Eating for Longevity: Unveiling the Secrets of Healthy Aging

HB Mostafa

Table of Contents

Chapter 1: Introduction to Healthy Aging

The Importance of Nutrition for Longevity

As we age, our bodies undergo various changes, and it becomes increasingly important to prioritize our health and well-being. One of the key factors in ensuring a long and healthy life is nutrition. The food we consume plays a vital role in determining our overall health and can significantly impact our longevity. In this subchapter, we will delve into the importance of nutrition for longevity, exploring the best diet and eating habits for healthy aging.

For aging adults and health-conscious individuals, understanding the significance of proper nutrition is essential. A well-balanced diet can provide the necessary nutrients, vitamins, and minerals that our bodies need to thrive. It can help prevent chronic diseases, boost the immune system, and support various bodily functions.

Research has shown that adopting a diet rich in fruits, vegetables, whole grains, lean proteins, and healthy fats can have profound effects on longevity. These foods are packed with antioxidants, which help combat oxidative stress and reduce the risk of age-related diseases such as heart disease, diabetes, and certain types of cancer.

Furthermore, nutrition plays a crucial role in maintaining a healthy weight. Excess weight can increase the risk of numerous health problems, including heart disease, stroke, and joint issues. By consuming a nutrient- dense, low-calorie diet, individuals can achieve and maintain a healthy weight, reducing the strain on their bodies and promoting longevity.

In addition to the types of food we consume, the timing and portion sizes also matter. Incorporating intermittent fasting or time-restricted eating can have significant benefits for longevity. These practices allow the body to rest and repair, promoting cellular regeneration and reducing the risk of age-related diseases.

Moreover, hydration is often overlooked but is equally important for healthy aging. Drinking an adequate amount of water throughout the day helps maintain proper bodily functions, supports digestion, and keeps the skin hydrated and youthful.

In conclusion, nutrition plays a pivotal role in determining our longevity. For aging adults and health-conscious individuals, adopting a well- balanced diet rich in fruits, vegetables, whole grains, lean proteins, and healthy fats is crucial. Additionally, incorporating intermittent fasting and staying properly hydrated can further enhance the benefits. By prioritizing nutrition, we can unlock the secrets of healthy aging and enjoy a long, vibrant life.

Understanding the Aging Process

As we journey through life, one inevitable aspect that we all encounter is the aging process. Aging is a natural phenomenon that affects every individual, and it is essential for aging adults and health-conscious individuals to understand the intricacies of this process. In this subchapter, we will delve deep into understanding the aging process and explore its impact on our overall health and well-being.

Aging is a complex and multifaceted process that involves the gradual decline of various bodily functions and systems. From a biological perspective, aging is characterized by a decrease in cell division, accumulation of cellular damage, and a decline in the body's ability to repair and regenerate itself. This process leads to a range of physical and cognitive changes, such as reduced muscle mass, diminished bone density, slower metabolism, and decreased cognitive function.

However, it is crucial to note that while aging is inevitable, its effects can be mitigated and managed through lifestyle choices, particularly in the realm of nutrition. Research has shown that adopting a healthy and balanced diet can significantly impact the aging process, promoting longevity and overall well-being.

Nutrition for longevity is about discovering the best diet and eating habits that support healthy aging. It involves consuming a wide variety of nutrient-rich foods, including fruits, vegetables, whole grains, lean proteins, and healthy fats. These foods provide essential vitamins, minerals, antioxidants, and phytochemicals that play a vital role in maintaining optimal health and combating age-related diseases.

Furthermore, understanding the impact of specific dietary components on the aging process can guide individuals in making informed choices. For instance, the consumption of antioxidant-rich foods like berries, leafy greens, and nuts can help reduce oxidative stress and inflammation, both of which are associated with the aging process.

In addition to a well-rounded diet, other lifestyle factors such as regular physical activity, stress management, and adequate sleep are also integral to healthy aging. Engaging in regular exercise helps improve cardiovascular health, maintain muscle strength, and enhance cognitive function. Managing stress through techniques like meditation and practicing good sleep hygiene ensures that the body can repair and regenerate effectively.

In conclusion, understanding the aging process is crucial for aging adults and health-conscious individuals seeking to promote healthy aging. By adopting a nutrition-focused approach and making conscious lifestyle choices, we can embrace the aging process gracefully and enjoy a life filled with vitality, resilience, and longevity.

The Benefits of Healthy Aging

As we journey through life, we all aspire to age gracefully and maintain our vitality and well-being. Aging is an inevitable part of life, but the good news is that healthy aging is within our reach. In this subchapter, we will delve into the numerous benefits of embracing a lifestyle that promotes healthy aging.

One of the primary benefits of healthy aging is the preservation of physical function. By adopting a nutritious diet and engaging in regular exercise, aging adults can maintain their strength, flexibility, and balance. This means fewer falls, a reduced risk of chronic diseases such as osteoporosis and arthritis, and the ability to continue enjoying an active lifestyle.

Another advantage of healthy aging is the preservation of cognitive function. The mind is a remarkable organ, and just like our bodies, it requires proper nourishment. Consuming a diet rich in brain-boosting nutrients, such as omega-3 fatty acids, antioxidants, and B vitamins, can help prevent cognitive decline and improve memory and focus. Additionally, engaging in mental exercises, such as puzzles or learning new skills, can keep the brain sharp and agile.

Healthy aging also promotes emotional well-being. As we age, we may face various challenges, including loss of loved ones, retirement, or health issues. However, by prioritizing self-care and adopting healthy habits, we can enhance our mental and emotional resilience. A balanced diet, regular exercise, and social connections can boost our mood, reduce stress, and promote a sense of purpose and fulfillment.

Furthermore, healthy aging is closely linked to longevity. By taking care of our bodies and minds, we increase our chances of enjoying a longer and more fulfilling life. Research has consistently shown that individuals who follow a healthy lifestyle, including a nutrient-dense diet and regular physical activity, tend to live longer and experience a higher quality of life.

In conclusion, healthy aging offers a multitude of benefits for aging adults and health-conscious individuals alike. By embracing a lifestyle that encompasses proper nutrition, regular exercise, and mental well-being, we can preserve physical function, enhance cognitive abilities, boost emotional health, and increase our chances of living a long and fulfilling life. Let's embark on this journey together, uncovering the secrets of healthy aging and discovering the best diet and eating habits for longevity.

Chapter 2: Exploring the Best Diet for Healthy Aging

The Basics of a Balanced Diet

In order to unlock the secrets of healthy aging, it is crucial to understand the basics of a balanced diet. As aging adults and health-conscious individuals, we must prioritize our nutrition for longevity. Our dietary choices play a vital role in promoting overall well-being and ensuring a healthy and fulfilling life.

A balanced diet consists of a combination of essential nutrients that provide our bodies with the fuel they need to function optimally. These nutrients include carbohydrates, proteins, fats, vitamins, minerals, and water. Each component plays a unique role in maintaining our health and vitality.

Carbohydrates are the primary source of energy for our bodies. It is important to choose complex carbohydrates such as whole grains, fruits, and vegetables over simple sugars found in processed foods. Complex carbohydrates provide sustained energy and are rich in fiber, which aids in digestion and prevents constipation.

Proteins are the building blocks of our bodies. They are essential for the growth, repair, and maintenance of tissues. Incorporating lean sources of protein such as fish, poultry, legumes, and nuts into our diet is crucial for maintaining muscle mass and supporting a strong immune system.

Healthy fats, such as those found in avocados, olive oil, and fatty fish, are essential for brain health, hormone production, and nutrient absorption. Including these fats in moderation can help reduce the risk of heart disease and improve cognitive function.

Vitamins and minerals are essential for various bodily functions. Incorporating a wide variety of fruits and vegetables into our diet ensures that we obtain a broad spectrum of these vital nutrients. Additionally, staying hydrated by drinking plenty of water promotes regular digestion, detoxification, and overall well-being.

In order to achieve a balanced diet, portion control is key. It is important to be mindful of serving sizes and avoid overeating. Additionally, incorporating regular exercise into our daily routine complements a balanced diet and promotes overall health and longevity.

Understanding the basics of a balanced diet is the first step towards healthy aging. By prioritizing nutrition for longevity, aging adults and health- conscious individuals can unlock the secrets to a fulfilling and vibrant life.

Essential Nutrients for Longevity

As we age, it becomes increasingly important to prioritize our health and make conscious choices that support healthy aging. One of the most crucial factors in maintaining our vitality and well-being is our diet. What we eat directly impacts our overall health, including our ability to live a long and fulfilling life. In this subchapter, we will explore the essential nutrients that can contribute to longevity, providing you with valuable insights into how to optimize your diet for healthy aging.

Protein, often referred to as the building block of life, is a fundamental nutrient for longevity. It plays a critical role in maintaining muscle mass, promoting tissue repair, and supporting a strong immune system. Aging adults should aim to include sources of lean protein, such as fish, poultry, legumes, and tofu, in their diet regularly.

Omega-3 fatty acids are another key nutrient for longevity. Found in fatty fish like salmon and mackerel, as well as flaxseeds and walnuts, these healthy fats have been shown to reduce inflammation, support brain health, and protect against heart disease. Including omega-3-rich foods in your diet can greatly contribute to a healthier, longer life.

Antioxidants are essential for combating the oxidative stress that occurs naturally as we age. These powerful compounds help protect our cells from damage caused by free radicals, reducing the risk of chronic diseases such as cancer and heart disease. Colorful fruits and vegetables, such as berries, leafy greens, and bell peppers, are excellent sources of antioxidants and should be incorporated into your daily meals.

Calcium and vitamin D are vital for maintaining bone health, especially as we age and become more susceptible to osteoporosis. Dairy products, fortified plant-based milk, and dark leafy greens are excellent sources of calcium, while exposure to sunlight and fortified foods can provide you with sufficient vitamin D.

Finally, fiber is a crucial nutrient for healthy aging. It aids in digestion, helps regulate blood sugar levels, and promotes heart health. Whole grains, fruits, vegetables, and legumes are all excellent sources of fiber that should be included in your diet.

By understanding the importance of these essential nutrients and incorporating them into your diet, you can promote healthy aging and increase your chances of living a long and fulfilling life. Remember, it's never too late to start prioritizing your health, and making conscious choices about what you eat can make all the difference in your journey towards longevity.

Foods to Include in Your Diet for Healthy Aging

As we age, maintaining good health becomes increasingly important. One of the key factors in promoting healthy aging is our diet. By making conscious choices about what we eat, we can support our bodies' natural aging processes and enhance overall well-being. In this subchapter, we will explore the top foods that should be included in your diet for healthy aging.

1. Colorful Fruits and Vegetables: Fill your plate with a variety of colorful fruits and vegetables. These nutrient-rich foods are packed with antioxidants, vitamins, and minerals that help fight off age-related diseases and promote overall vitality. Aim for at least five servings per day, including leafy greens, berries, citrus fruits, and cruciferous vegetables like broccoli and cauliflower.

2. Lean Protein: Incorporate lean protein sources such as fish, poultry, beans, and tofu into your meals. Protein is essential for maintaining muscle mass, supporting bone health, and promoting a healthy immune system. Choose lean cuts of meat and opt for plant-based protein sources on alternate days to reduce saturated fat intake.

3. Whole Grains: Swap refined grains for whole grains like quinoa, brown rice, and whole wheat bread. These complex carbohydrates provide sustained energy, fiber, and important nutrients. They also

promote digestive health and help manage weight, reducing the risk of age-related conditions like diabetes and heart disease.

4. Healthy Fats: Include sources of healthy fats in your diet, such as avocados, nuts, seeds, and olive oil. These fats are beneficial for brain health, reducing inflammation, and supporting heart health. However, moderation is key, as they are calorie-dense. Aim for small portions to maintain a balanced diet.

5. Dairy or Dairy Alternatives: Incorporate low-fat dairy products or plant- based alternatives fortified with calcium and vitamin D. These nutrients are crucial for maintaining strong bones and reducing the risk of osteoporosis. Yogurt, milk, and fortified plant-based milk are excellent choices.

6. Hydration: Don't forget the importance of staying hydrated. Aim for at least 8-10 glasses of water per day, and include herbal teas, soups, and fruits with high water content to meet your hydration needs.

By including these foods in your diet, you can support healthy aging and enhance your overall well-being. Remember, it's not just about individual foods, but also about maintaining a balanced and varied diet. Consult a registered dietitian or healthcare professional for personalized advice tailored to your specific needs. Eating well is a key ingredient for a long and healthy life.

Chapter 3: The Power of Anti-Aging Foods

Antioxidants: Nature's Anti-Aging Agents

In the quest for healthy aging, one cannot underestimate the power of antioxidants. These remarkable compounds, found abundantly in nature, are nature's anti-aging agents. They play a crucial role in combating the harmful effects of free radicals and oxidative stress, which are major contributors to the aging process. In this subchapter, we will delve into the world of antioxidants and explore how they can help us slow down the aging clock and achieve optimal health.

Firstly, let's understand what antioxidants are. Simply put, antioxidants are substances that can neutralize free radicals, unstable molecules that can damage cells and DNA. Free radicals are produced naturally in our bodies as a result of metabolic processes, but they can also be generated by external factors such as pollution, radiation, and smoking. When left unchecked, free radicals can wreak havoc on our bodies, leading to chronic inflammation, cellular damage, and accelerated aging.

The good news is that antioxidants can help counteract these harmful effects. By donating an electron to the free radicals, antioxidants effectively neutralize them, preventing them from causing further damage. Furthermore, antioxidants have been shown to possess anti- inflammatory properties, which can help reduce the risk of chronic diseases associated with aging, such as heart disease, diabetes, and cancer.

So, where can we find these powerful antioxidants? Fortunately, they are present in a wide variety of foods, particularly fruits, vegetables, nuts, and seeds. For instance, colorful fruits and vegetables like berries, spinach, kale, and tomatoes are rich in antioxidants such as vitamins A, C, and E, as well as plant compounds like flavonoids and carotenoids. Other excellent sources of antioxidants include green tea, dark chocolate, and spices like turmeric and cinnamon.

Incorporating these antioxidant-rich foods into our diet is essential for healthy aging. However, it's important to note that getting a variety of antioxidants from different sources is key. Each antioxidant has its unique benefits, and by consuming a diverse range of foods, we can ensure we reap the full spectrum of antioxidant power.

In conclusion, antioxidants are nature's gift to us in the fight against aging. By incorporating antioxidant-rich foods into our diet, we can protect our cells from oxidative damage, reduce inflammation, and promote healthy aging. So, let's embrace the power of antioxidants and make them a foundational part of our nutrition for longevity journey.

Superfoods for Longevity

Subchapter: Superfoods for Longevity
Introduction:

In our quest for healthy aging, nutrition plays a pivotal role. The foods we consume can either promote longevity or accelerate the aging process. In this subchapter, we will delve into the world of superfoods for longevity.

These nutrient-dense powerhouses are packed with antioxidants, vitamins, minerals, and various other compounds that can support healthy aging. By incorporating these superfoods into your diet, you can nourish your body and enhance your overall well-being.

1. Blueberries:

Blueberries are often hailed as the king of superfoods. Packed with antioxidants, these tiny berries can help combat inflammation and oxidative stress, two major factors in aging. They are also rich in fiber, which aids digestion and supports heart health.

2. Leafy Greens:

Leafy greens such as spinach, kale, and Swiss chard are nutritional powerhouses. Loaded with vitamins A, C, and K, along with antioxidants and fiber, they can help protect against age-related diseases. These greens also contain high levels of folate, which supports brain health and cognitive function.

3. Fatty Fish:

Fish like salmon, mackerel, and sardines are abundant in omega-3 fatty acids. These healthy fats have been linked to a reduced risk of heart disease, cognitive decline, and inflammation. Incorporating fatty fish into your diet can support brain health and promote longevity.

4. Turmeric:

Turmeric is a vibrant spice commonly used in Indian cuisine. It contains a compound called curcumin, which has potent anti-inflammatory and antioxidant properties. Curcumin has been associated with a decreased risk of chronic diseases, including heart disease and certain types of cancer.

5. Nuts and Seeds:

Almonds, walnuts, flaxseeds, and chia seeds are excellent sources of healthy fats, fiber, and essential nutrients. These foods can help reduce inflammation, support brain health, and lower the risk of heart disease. Including a handful of nuts and seeds in your daily diet can be beneficial for healthy aging.

Conclusion:

Embracing a diet rich in superfoods can be a game-changer for healthy aging. Incorporating blueberries, leafy greens, fatty fish, turmeric, nuts, and seeds into your daily meals can provide your body with the necessary nutrients to thrive. By making these superfoods a part of your nutrition for longevity, you can unlock the secrets to healthy aging and enjoy a vibrant, fulfilling life for years to come.

Incorporating Anti-Aging Foods into Your Meals

As we age, it becomes increasingly important to prioritize our health and well-being. One of the most effective ways to do this is by paying attention to what we eat. Nutrition plays a critical role in healthy aging, and incorporating anti-aging foods into our meals can make a significant difference in our overall well-being.

Anti-aging foods are packed with antioxidants, vitamins, minerals, and other essential nutrients that combat the damage caused by free radicals and promote a youthful, vibrant appearance. These foods not only help us maintain a healthy weight but also reduce the risk of chronic diseases such as heart disease, diabetes, and certain types of cancer.

So, what are these magical anti-aging foods? Well, they are actually quite common and can easily be incorporated into our everyday meals. Here are some key examples:

1. Berries: Blueberries, strawberries, and raspberries are rich in antioxidants that protect our cells from oxidative stress and inflammation. They also contain a high amount of fiber, which aids digestion and promotes a healthy gut.

2. Leafy greens: Spinach, kale, and Swiss chard are packed with vitamins A, C, and K, as well as folate and iron. These nutrients help maintain healthy bones, boost the immune system, and provide anti-inflammatory benefits.

3. Fatty fish: Salmon, mackerel, and sardines are excellent sources of omega-3 fatty acids, which are essential for brain health and reducing the risk of age-related cognitive decline. They also provide high-quality protein, which aids in muscle repair and maintenance.

4. Nuts and seeds: Almonds, walnuts, flaxseeds, and chia seeds are rich in healthy fats, fiber, and essential minerals. They provide a satisfying crunch to meals and can help lower cholesterol levels and reduce the risk of heart disease.

5. Whole grains: Quinoa, brown rice, and whole wheat bread are excellent sources of complex carbohydrates, fiber, and B-vitamins. These foods help regulate blood sugar levels, promote healthy digestion, and provide long- lasting energy.

Incorporating these anti-aging foods into our meals is easier than it may seem. We can start by adding a handful of berries to our morning cereal, incorporating leafy greens into our lunchtime salads, and replacing refined grains with whole grains for dinner. Small changes like these can have a significant impact on our health and vitality as we age.

Remember, healthy aging is a lifelong journey, and adopting a diet rich in anti-aging foods is an essential step towards achieving longevity and overall well-being. So, let's make conscious choices when it comes to our meals and embrace the power of nutrition for a healthy, vibrant future.

Chapter 4: Creating a Longevity Meal Plan

Identifying Your Nutritional Needs

In the journey towards healthy aging, one of the most crucial aspects to consider is nutrition. As aging adults and health-conscious individuals, understanding and identifying your nutritional needs becomes imperative to ensure a vibrant and energetic life. This subchapter aims to enlighten you about the factors that influence your nutritional requirements and how to tailor your diet accordingly.

As we age, our bodies undergo various physiological changes that can impact our nutritional needs. Factors such as decreased metabolism, changes in body composition, and a decline in organ function necessitate adjustments in our dietary choices. It is essential to focus on nutrient- dense foods that provide the necessary vitamins, minerals, and antioxidants to support our overall health and combat age-related ailments.

The first step in identifying your nutritional needs is to assess your own individual requirements. Every person is unique, and factors like gender, age, weight, and activity level play a significant role in determining your nutrient intake. Consulting with a registered dietitian or a healthcare professional can provide valuable insights into your specific nutritional needs and help you formulate a personalized dietary plan.

Furthermore, understanding the concept of macronutrients and micronutrients is vital. Macronutrients, including carbohydrates, proteins, and fats, form the foundation of our diet and provide us with energy.

Balancing these macronutrients according to your needs is crucial to maintain a healthy weight and support bodily functions. Micronutrients, such as vitamins and minerals, are equally important and contribute to various bodily processes, including immune function, bone health, and cognitive performance. Incorporating a wide variety of fruits, vegetables, whole grains, lean proteins, and healthy fats into your diet ensures an adequate intake of these essential micronutrients.

Another aspect to consider when identifying your nutritional needs is any specific health conditions or concerns you may have. Certain medical conditions, such as diabetes, heart disease, or osteoporosis, may require dietary modifications to manage symptoms effectively. Additionally, taking into account any food allergies or intolerances is crucial to ensure your nutritional needs are met without compromising your well-being.

In conclusion, identifying your nutritional needs is a

fundamental step towards healthy aging. By understanding your individual requirements, focusing on nutrient-dense foods, and considering any specific health concerns, you can create a dietary plan that supports your overall well- being and longevity. Remember, consulting with a healthcare professional or registered dietitian is invaluable in this process, as they can provide personalized guidance tailored to your unique needs. Embrace the power of nutrition and embark on a journey towards a vibrant and fulfilling life.

Designing a Balanced Meal Plan

A key factor in promoting healthy aging is maintaining a well-balanced diet. As we age, our nutritional needs change, and it becomes crucial to ensure that our bodies receive the necessary nutrients to support overall health and vitality. In this subchapter, we will explore the principles of designing a balanced meal plan that caters specifically to the needs of aging adults and health-conscious individuals.

The first step in creating a balanced meal plan is to focus on whole, nutrient-dense foods. These include fruits, vegetables, whole grains, lean proteins, and healthy fats. By incorporating a variety of these foods into your diet, you can ensure that you are getting a wide range of essential vitamins, minerals, and antioxidants.

Portion control is another important aspect of a balanced meal plan. As we age, our metabolism slows down, and it becomes easier to gain weight. By practicing portion control, you can maintain a healthy weight and reduce the risk of chronic diseases such as heart disease and diabetes. A useful strategy is to use smaller plates and bowls and to listen to your body's hunger and fullness cues.

Furthermore, it is essential to pay attention to the quality of the carbohydrates you consume. Opt for complex carbohydrates, such as whole grains, legumes, and vegetables, over simple carbohydrates like refined grains and sugars. Complex carbohydrates provide sustained energy, stabilize blood sugar levels, and promote digestive health.

Protein intake is also crucial for healthy aging. Include lean sources of protein in your meal plan, such as fish, poultry, beans, and nuts. Protein aids in maintaining muscle mass, supports immune function, and repairs tissues. Aim to incorporate protein into every meal and snack.

Lastly, do not forget about hydration. Older adults are more prone to dehydration, which can lead to various health issues. Make sure to drink plenty of water throughout the day and include hydrating foods such as fruits and vegetables in your meal plan.

Designing a balanced meal plan that focuses on whole, nutrient-dense foods, portion control, quality carbohydrates, protein, and hydration is essential for healthy aging. By adopting these principles, you can optimize your nutrition, support healthy aging, and enhance overall well-being.

Remember, it is never too late to make positive changes to your diet and reap the benefits of healthy eating.

Meal Prepping for Healthy Aging

Meal prepping is a valuable tool for aging adults and health-conscious individuals who are determined to maintain their well-being and vitality as they age. With proper nutrition, we can unlock the secrets of healthy aging and promote longevity.

Nutrition for longevity plays a crucial role in healthy aging. The food we consume directly impacts our energy levels, cognitive function, and overall physical health. By adopting meal prepping techniques, we can ensure that we have access to nutritious meals throughout the week, even when our schedules become hectic.

One of the key benefits of meal prepping is the ability to control the ingredients and portion sizes of our meals. This allows us to focus on consuming nutrient-dense foods and avoiding excessive calories, sodium, and unhealthy fats. By planning and preparing our meals in advance, we can make conscious choices about incorporating a variety of fruits, vegetables, whole grains, lean proteins, and healthy fats into our diet.

Meal prepping also offers the opportunity to experiment with new recipes and flavors. Aging adults can explore different cuisines and incorporate foods that they may not have tried before. By diversifying our meals, we can benefit from a wide range of essential nutrients and antioxidants, which can help protect our bodies against age-related diseases and promote healthy aging.

In addition to promoting a nutritious diet, meal prepping can also save time and money. By dedicating a few hours each week to meal prepping, we can streamline our cooking process and avoid the temptation of ordering takeout or relying on processed foods. With pre-prepared meals ready to go, we can resist the temptation to make unhealthy food choices when time is limited or when we're feeling fatigued.

To get started with meal prepping, it's essential to plan your meals in advance. Set aside time each week to create a meal plan, taking into consideration your nutritional needs and preferences. Make a shopping list and stock up on fresh ingredients. Choose recipes that can be easily prepared in large quantities and stored in individual portions. Invest in airtight containers and label them with the date to ensure freshness.

By embracing meal prepping for healthy aging, we can take control of our nutrition, promote longevity, and enjoy the benefits of a balanced diet.

With a little planning and preparation, we can ensure that our meals are not only delicious but also support our health and well-being as we age.

Chapter 5: Eating Habits for Longevity

Mindful Eating: The Key to Healthy Aging

In today's fast-paced world, where convenience often trumps health, it is crucial for aging adults and health-conscious individuals to embrace the practice of mindful eating. This subchapter will delve into the significance of mindful eating as the key to healthy aging, providing valuable insights into how it can positively impact our overall well-being and longevity.

As we age, our bodies undergo various changes that necessitate a more mindful approach to our eating habits. Metabolism slows down, nutrient absorption becomes less efficient, and the risk of chronic diseases increases. However, by adopting mindful eating practices, we can combat these challenges and enjoy a healthier and more vibrant life.

Mindful eating involves being fully present and engaged in the act of eating, paying attention to our body's hunger and fullness cues, and savoring each bite. By doing so, we can better regulate our portion sizes, make healthier food choices, and cultivate a deeper connection with the nourishing power of food.

One of the primary benefits of mindful eating for healthy aging is improved digestion. By slowing down and savoring

each bite, we allow our bodies to properly break down and absorb nutrients, reducing the likelihood of digestive issues such as bloating and indigestion.
Additionally, mindful eating promotes weight management by preventing overeating and promoting a healthier relationship with food.

Furthermore, mindful eating has a positive impact on our mental and emotional well-being. By being fully present during meals, we can truly enjoy the sensory experience of eating, enhancing our satisfaction and reducing the need for emotional eating. This practice also helps to alleviate stress and anxiety, which are common challenges faced by aging adults.

Lastly, mindful eating allows us to make informed and conscious food choices. By paying attention to the nutritional content and quality of the foods we consume, we can ensure that our bodies receive the necessary nutrients for healthy aging. This includes incorporating a variety of whole foods, such as fruits, vegetables, whole grains, and lean proteins, while minimizing processed and sugary foods.

In conclusion, mindful eating is a powerful tool for aging adults and health-conscious individuals seeking to optimize their well-being and promote healthy aging. By adopting this practice, we can improve digestion, manage weight, enhance mental and emotional well-being, and make conscious food choices. Let us embark on this mindful eating journey and unlock the secrets to healthy aging through the power of nourishing our bodies and minds.

Portion Control for Longevity

In our quest for healthy aging, it's essential to pay attention not only to the quality of food we consume but also to the quantity. Portion control plays a vital role in maintaining a healthy weight, preventing chronic diseases, and ultimately promoting longevity. By understanding the importance of portion control and implementing it into our daily lives, we can unlock the secrets of healthy aging.

Portion control refers to the practice of eating the right amount of food to meet our body's nutritional needs, without overindulging. As we age, our metabolism slows down, making it easier to gain weight. However, by practicing portion control, we can maintain a healthy weight and reduce the risk of obesity-related health issues such as heart disease, diabetes, and certain cancers.

One effective method of portion control is using visual cues. Instead of relying solely on measuring cups or scales, visualize portion sizes based on familiar objects. For example, a serving of meat should be about the size of a deck of cards, while a cup of vegetables is roughly the size of a tennis ball. By training our eyes to estimate portion sizes, we can better control our intake.

Another useful strategy is to listen to our body's hunger and fullness cues. Aging adults often find their appetites decrease, and they may not need as much food as they used to. Paying attention to these signals helps prevent overeating and allows us to eat until we are satisfied, rather than stuffed.
Eating slowly and mindfully can also aid in recognizing these cues and enjoying our meals more fully.

Additionally, it's important to be mindful of portion control when dining out or ordering takeout. Restaurant portions tend to be larger than what is necessary, leading to overeating. Consider sharing a meal with a friend or opting for an appetizer or smaller portion from the menu. Taking home leftovers for another meal is also a great way to practice portion control.

By incorporating portion control into our daily eating habits, we can ensure we are fueling our bodies with the right amount of nutrients, while also preventing excessive calorie intake. This, in turn, promotes healthy aging and reduces the risk of chronic diseases associated with weight gain.
Remember, it's not just what we eat, but how much we eat that matters for longevity.

Hydration and its Impact on Aging

As we age, it becomes increasingly important to prioritize our overall health and well-being. One crucial aspect that often goes unnoticed is hydration. Many aging adults and health-conscious individuals may not realize the significant role that adequate hydration plays in healthy aging. In this subchapter, we will delve into the various ways in which hydration impacts the aging process and uncover the secrets to maintaining optimal hydration levels for longevity.

Water is the elixir of life, and it serves as the foundation for numerous bodily functions. Staying hydrated is essential for maintaining healthy skin, promoting digestion, regulating body temperature, and supporting joint health. However, as we age, our bodies become less efficient at retaining water, making it even more crucial to prioritize hydration.

Dehydration is a common issue among aging adults and can lead to numerous health complications. It can exacerbate existing conditions such as arthritis, increase the risk of urinary tract infections, and even impair cognitive function. By understanding the importance of hydration, we can take proactive steps to combat these issues and promote healthy aging.

In addition to drinking water, incorporating hydrating foods into our diets is essential. Fruits and vegetables with high water content, such as watermelon, cucumber, and oranges, can provide an excellent source of hydration. Furthermore, avoiding excessive consumption of dehydrating substances like caffeine and alcohol is crucial for maintaining optimal hydration levels.

To ensure proper hydration, it is essential to listen to our bodies and recognize the signs of dehydration. Thirst is not always an accurate indicator of hydration status, especially for aging adults. Therefore, it is recommended to establish a routine of regular fluid intake throughout the day, even if thirst is not present.

In conclusion, understanding the impact of hydration on aging is vital for aging adults and health-conscious individuals. By prioritizing hydration, we can promote healthy aging, combat age-related health issues, and enhance overall well-being. Incorporating hydrating foods, avoiding dehydrating substances, and establishing a regular fluid intake routine are key steps towards maintaining optimal hydration levels for longevity.

Remember, water is the elixir of life, and by giving our bodies what they need, we can unlock the secrets to healthy aging and longevity.

Chapter 6: Addressing Common Health Conditions in Aging Adults

Heart Health and Longevity

In this subchapter, we will delve into the crucial connection between heart health and longevity. As aging adults and health-conscious individuals, it is essential to prioritize the well-being of our cardiovascular system, as it plays a vital role in our overall longevity and quality of life. By adopting proper nutrition and lifestyle habits, we can significantly enhance our heart health and ultimately extend our years of healthy aging.

The first step towards promoting heart health is understanding the impact of our dietary choices. A diet rich in fruits, vegetables, whole grains, and lean proteins can provide the necessary nutrients to support a healthy heart. Incorporating foods that are low in saturated fats and cholesterol and high in fiber can help to lower the risk of heart disease, a leading cause of mortality among aging adults. Furthermore, reducing sodium intake can help maintain healthy blood pressure levels and prevent the onset of hypertension.

In addition to a balanced diet, regular physical activity is another crucial aspect of maintaining a healthy heart. Engaging in moderate-intensity exercises such as brisk walking, swimming, or cycling for at least 30 minutes a day can strengthen the heart muscle, improve blood circulation, and reduce the risk of cardiovascular diseases. It is important to consult with a healthcare professional before starting any exercise regimen, especially if you have pre-existing heart conditions.

Furthermore, managing stress levels is paramount for heart health and longevity. Chronic stress can contribute to the development of heart disease and other health problems. Incorporating stress-reducing techniques such as meditation, deep breathing exercises, or engaging in hobbies can promote a sense of calm and overall well-being.

Lastly, regular check-ups and screenings are essential for monitoring heart health. Aging adults should schedule routine appointments with their healthcare providers to assess blood pressure, cholesterol levels, and overall cardiovascular health. Early detection and intervention can significantly improve outcomes and prevent potential complications.

In conclusion, prioritizing heart health is crucial for aging adults and health-conscious individuals looking to enhance their longevity. By adopting a balanced diet, engaging in regular physical activity, managing stress levels, and seeking regular medical check-ups, we can significantly reduce the risk of heart disease and promote healthy aging. Remember, a healthy heart lays the foundation for a long and fulfilling life.

Maintaining Healthy Bones and Joints

Subchapter: Maintaining Healthy Bones and Joints
As we age, maintaining healthy bones and joints becomes crucial for overall well-being and longevity. Our bones provide structural support to our bodies, while our joints enable movement and flexibility. In order to preserve and strengthen these vital components of our musculoskeletal system, it is important to adopt a holistic approach that includes proper nutrition and lifestyle choices.

Nutrition plays a pivotal role in maintaining healthy bones and joints. Calcium and Vitamin D are essential nutrients that promote bone health. Aging adults should aim to consume calcium-rich foods such as dairy products, leafy greens, and fortified plant-based milk. Additionally, getting enough sunlight exposure or taking Vitamin D supplements is beneficial for calcium absorption. Magnesium, found in nuts, seeds, and whole grains, also contributes to bone health by enhancing calcium absorption and bone density.

Another crucial nutrient for joint health is Omega-3 fatty acids. These healthy fats can be found in fatty fish like salmon, mackerel, and sardines, as well as flaxseeds and walnuts.

Omega-3 fatty acids possess anti- inflammatory properties, which can help reduce joint pain and inflammation associated with conditions like arthritis.

Incorporating a variety of fruits and vegetables into your diet is also important for maintaining healthy bones and joints. These colorful plant foods provide antioxidants that protect against cellular damage, promoting overall joint health. Additionally, they contain essential vitamins and minerals that support bone density, such as Vitamin C, Vitamin K, and potassium.

While proper nutrition is crucial, it is equally important to engage in regular physical activity to maintain healthy bones and joints. Weight- bearing exercises, such as walking, jogging, or dancing, help strengthen bones and improve joint flexibility. Strength-training exercises, like lifting weights or using resistance bands, can also help build and maintain muscle strength, which provides support to the joints.

Furthermore, maintaining a healthy weight is essential for bone and joint health. Excess weight puts additional stress on our joints, increasing the risk of joint problems and conditions such as osteoarthritis. By adopting a balanced diet and engaging in regular exercise, we can achieve and maintain a healthy weight, reducing the strain on our bones and joints.

In conclusion, maintaining healthy bones and joints is crucial for aging adults and health-conscious individuals. By incorporating calcium, Vitamin D, Omega-3 fatty acids, and a variety of fruits and vegetables into our diets, we can support bone density and joint health. Regular physical activity, including weight-bearing exercises and strength training, is also essential for maintaining healthy bones and joints. By adopting these lifestyle choices, we can enhance our overall well-being and promote healthy aging.

Cognitive Function and Aging

As we age, it is natural for our bodies and minds to undergo certain changes. One area that often raises concerns among aging adults and health-conscious individuals is cognitive function. Cognitive function refers to our ability to think, learn, remember, and make decisions. It encompasses processes such as attention, perception, memory, language, and problem-solving. While some decline in cognitive function is a normal part of aging, there are ways to support and maintain healthy brain function as we grow older.

Nutrition plays a crucial role in maintaining cognitive function and promoting healthy aging. Research has shown that certain nutrients can enhance brain health and protect against age-related cognitive decline. Antioxidants, found in fruits and vegetables, help reduce oxidative stress and inflammation, which can contribute to cognitive decline. Omega-3 fatty acids, commonly found in fish and nuts, are essential for brain health and have been shown to improve memory and cognitive performance. B vitamins, particularly vitamin B12, are important for maintaining healthy brain function and can be obtained through foods such as eggs, meat, and dairy products.

In addition to these specific nutrients, adopting a healthy eating pattern is essential for supporting cognitive function as we age. The Mediterranean diet, for example, has been widely studied and is associated with a reduced risk of cognitive decline and dementia. This eating pattern emphasizes fruits, vegetables, whole grains, legumes, fish, and olive oil while limiting red meat, processed foods, and sugary beverages. The DASH (Dietary Approaches to Stop Hypertension) diet, which focuses on fruits, vegetables, low-fat dairy products, and lean proteins, has also been linked to better cognitive function.

Incorporating these dietary recommendations into your daily life can have significant benefits for cognitive function and healthy aging. However, nutrition is just one piece of the puzzle. Regular physical activity, mental stimulation, social engagement, and quality sleep are also vital for maintaining cognitive function. It is important to engage in activities that challenge the brain, such as puzzles, reading, or learning a new skill.

Building and maintaining strong social connections, as well as getting enough restorative sleep, are also essential for overall brain health.

In conclusion, cognitive function and aging are interconnected, and nutrition plays a crucial role in maintaining brain health as we grow older. By adopting a healthy eating pattern rich in antioxidants, omega-3 fatty acids, and B vitamins, such as the Mediterranean or DASH diet, individuals can support cognitive function and promote healthy aging. However, it is important to remember that nutrition is just one aspect of a comprehensive approach to brain health. Engaging in physical activity, mental stimulation, social connections, and quality sleep are also essential for maintaining cognitive function and overall well-being as we age.

Chapter 7: Supplements for Healthy Aging

Understanding the Role of Supplements

In the pursuit of healthy aging, nutrition plays a vital role. As aging adults and health-conscious individuals, we understand the significance of consuming a well-balanced diet to support our overall well-being.

However, even with the best diet and eating habits, it can be challenging to obtain all the essential nutrients our bodies need solely from food. This is where supplements come into play.

Supplements are a valuable addition to our daily routine, as they provide the necessary nutrients that may be lacking in our diet. While they should never replace a healthy diet, they can certainly complement it.

Understanding the role of supplements is crucial to optimizing our health and longevity.

One of the key benefits of supplements is their ability to fill in nutritional gaps. As we age, our bodies may have difficulty absorbing certain nutrients from food, leading to deficiencies. For example, calcium and vitamin D are essential for maintaining strong bones, but they may become harder to absorb with age. In such cases, supplements can ensure that we meet our daily requirements and support bone health.

Another important role of supplements is to provide additional support for specific health concerns. As aging adults, we may face various health challenges, such as joint pain, cognitive decline, or heart health issues.

Certain supplements, such as glucosamine for joint health, omega-3 fatty acids for brain function, or CoQ10 for cardiovascular health, can be beneficial in addressing these concerns and promoting overall well-being.

Additionally, supplements can act as antioxidants, protecting our bodies from the damage caused by free radicals. Antioxidants, such as vitamins C and E, selenium, or resveratrol, help fight oxidative stress and reduce the risk of chronic diseases associated with aging, including heart disease and certain cancers.

However, it is important to approach supplements with caution. Not all supplements are created equal, and their efficacy can vary. It is crucial to consult with a healthcare professional or a registered dietitian before incorporating any new supplements into our regimen. They can assess our specific needs, determine potential interactions with medications, and recommend the most appropriate and effective options for our individual circumstances.

In conclusion, supplements play a significant role in supporting our health and longevity as aging adults and health-conscious individuals. They can fill nutritional gaps, provide targeted support for specific health concerns, and act as antioxidants to combat aging-related damage. However, it is essential to approach supplements with knowledge and seek professional guidance to ensure their safety and effectiveness. By understanding the role of supplements and incorporating them appropriately, we can optimize our nutrition for longevity and unveil the secrets of healthy aging.

Key Supplements for Longevity

In the pursuit of healthy aging, nutrition plays a crucial role. While a well- balanced diet is essential, there are certain key supplements that can further enhance longevity and well-being. These supplements provide the body with vital nutrients that may not be obtained in sufficient quantities through diet alone. In this subchapter, we will explore the top supplements for longevity and their benefits for aging adults and health-conscious individuals.

1. Omega-3 Fatty Acids: Omega-3s are essential for brain health, heart function, and reducing inflammation. Found in fatty fish like salmon, mackerel, and sardines, omega-3s can also be taken in supplement form. They have been shown to improve cognitive function, support cardiovascular health, and reduce the risk of chronic diseases such as Alzheimer's and heart disease.

2. Vitamin D: Known as the sunshine vitamin, vitamin D is crucial for bone health, immune function, and reducing the risk of chronic diseases. Aging adults often have reduced sun exposure and may require supplementation. Vitamin D supplements have been linked to a lower risk of osteoporosis, depression, and certain types of cancer.

3. Coenzyme Q10 (CoQ10): CoQ10 is a naturally occurring compound that plays a vital role in energy production within cells.

As we age, our CoQ10 levels decline, impacting overall energy levels. Supplementing with CoQ10 can help boost cellular energy production, support heart health, and reduce the risk of age-related conditions such as Parkinson's disease.

4. Probiotics: Gut health becomes increasingly important as we age. Probiotics are beneficial bacteria that promote a healthy gut microbiome. They help improve digestion, strengthen the immune system, and enhance nutrient absorption. Aging adults can benefit from taking probiotic supplements or consuming fermented foods like yogurt and sauerkraut.

5. Resveratrol: Resveratrol is a powerful antioxidant found in red wine, grapes, and berries. It has been studied for its potential anti-aging effects, including the activation of longevity genes. Resveratrol supplements may help reduce inflammation, protect against age-related cognitive decline, and support heart health.

While these supplements can offer numerous benefits for healthy aging, it's important to consult a healthcare professional before starting any new supplement regimen. They can assess individual needs, potential interactions with medications, and recommend the appropriate dosages.

Remember, supplements should never replace a nutrient-rich diet. They are meant to complement a healthy lifestyle and support optimal longevity. By incorporating these key supplements into your routine, you can take proactive steps towards aging gracefully and enjoying a vibrant, healthy life.

Consultation and Evaluation Before Taking Supplements

As we age, it becomes increasingly important to take care of our bodies and provide them with the necessary nutrients for healthy aging. While a balanced diet rich in fruits, vegetables, whole grains, and lean proteins should be the foundation of our nutrition, sometimes it may be necessary to supplement our diet with additional nutrients. However, before embarking on any supplement regimen, it is essential to consult with a healthcare professional and evaluate our individual needs.

Consultation with a healthcare professional is crucial for several reasons. Firstly, they can assess our current health status and identify any deficiencies or imbalances in our diet. They can also evaluate any pre- existing medical conditions or medications that may interact with certain supplements. This personalized assessment allows for tailored recommendations that align with our specific needs and goals.

Furthermore, a healthcare professional can guide us through the overwhelming world of supplements, helping us differentiate between evidence-based products and those lacking scientific support. With an abundance of supplements available on the market, it is easy to fall prey to misleading claims and ineffective products. A consultation will ensure that we make informed choices based on our individual circumstances.

Evaluation before taking supplements also involves understanding the potential risks and benefits associated with each supplement. While some nutrients are generally safe for consumption, others may have adverse effects when taken in excessive amounts or in combination with certain medications. By discussing our medical history and current health status with a healthcare professional, we can identify any potential risks and determine the appropriate dosage and form of supplementation.

Moreover, evaluation should also extend to the quality and reliability of the supplement itself. Not all supplements are created equal, and their potency and purity can vary significantly. It is important to choose products from reputable manufacturers that adhere to strict quality control standards. A healthcare professional can recommend trusted brands and help navigate the often-confusing world of supplement labels and ingredients.

In conclusion, before incorporating supplements into our

diet, consultation and evaluation with a healthcare professional are essential steps. They can provide personalized guidance, ensuring that we choose the right supplements for our individual needs and reduce the risk of adverse effects. By taking this proactive approach, we can optimize our nutrition for longevity and healthy aging, keeping our bodies nourished and vibrant for years to come.

Chapter 8: Lifestyle Factors for Longevity

Exercise and its Impact on Aging

Regular physical activity is an essential component of healthy aging. As we age, our bodies undergo numerous changes, including a decrease in muscle mass, a decline in bone density, and a reduction in cardiovascular fitness. However, engaging in regular exercise can help mitigate these age- related changes and improve overall health and well-being.

One of the most notable benefits of exercise for aging adults is its positive impact on muscle strength and endurance. Strength training exercises, such as weightlifting or resistance training, can help build and maintain muscle mass, which can help combat age-related muscle loss, also known as sarcopenia. By preserving muscle mass, older adults can improve their mobility, balance, and independence, reducing the risk of falls and injuries.

Exercise also plays a crucial role in maintaining bone health, particularly in preventing osteoporosis. Weight-bearing exercises, such as walking, jogging, or dancing, stimulate the bones to become stronger and denser. This can reduce the risk of fractures and improve overall bone health, which tends to decline with age.

Furthermore, regular exercise has a significant impact on cardiovascular health. It can help lower blood pressure, reduce the risk of heart disease, and improve overall cardiovascular fitness. Engaging in aerobic activities, such as swimming, cycling, or brisk walking, can enhance heart and lung function, increase stamina, and improve circulation. This, in turn, can lead to a reduced risk of chronic diseases and an increased quality of life.

Exercise has also been shown to have positive effects on cognitive function and mental health. Physical activity increases blood flow to the brain, promoting the growth of new neurons and improving cognitive abilities, including memory and attention. Additionally, exercise releases endorphins, the body's natural mood boosters, which can help alleviate symptoms of depression and anxiety commonly experienced by aging adults.

Incorporating exercise into a daily routine doesn't have to be complicated or time-consuming. Even simple activities like walking, gardening, or yoga can provide significant health benefits. It's important to choose activities that are enjoyable and sustainable to ensure adherence and consistency.

In conclusion, exercise has a profound impact on aging,

offering numerous physical and mental health benefits. By engaging in regular physical activity, aging adults can improve muscle strength, maintain bone density, enhance cardiovascular health, and boost cognitive function. Exercise is a powerful tool for healthy aging, and incorporating it into our lives can lead to a longer, healthier, and more fulfilling life.

Stress Management for Healthy Aging

In the fast-paced world we live in today, stress has become an inevitable part of our daily lives. However, as aging adults and health-conscious individuals, it is crucial to prioritize stress management in order to maintain our overall well-being. In this subchapter, we will explore effective strategies to manage stress and promote healthy aging.

First and foremost, it is important to understand that chronic stress can have detrimental effects on our physical and mental health. It can weaken our immune system, accelerate the aging process, and increase the risk of various diseases. Therefore, finding ways to effectively manage stress becomes even more crucial as we age.

One of the most effective stress management techniques is regular physical activity. Engaging in activities such as walking, swimming, yoga, or tai chi not only helps to release endorphins, the feel-good hormones, but also improves cardiovascular health and enhances overall well-being.

Additionally, regular exercise promotes better sleep, which further aids in stress reduction.

Another important aspect of stress management is maintaining a healthy and balanced diet. Consuming nutrient-dense foods, such as fruits, vegetables, whole grains, lean proteins, and healthy fats, can provide the necessary nutrients to support our body's stress response system. It is also important to limit the intake of processed foods, sugary snacks, and caffeine, as they can exacerbate feelings of stress and anxiety.

In addition to exercise and nutrition, incorporating relaxation techniques into our daily routine can significantly reduce stress levels. Practices such as deep breathing exercises, meditation, mindfulness, and engaging in hobbies or activities that bring joy and relaxation can help to calm the mind and promote a sense of peace and well-being.

Furthermore, maintaining a strong support system is vital for stress management. Surrounding ourselves with positive and supportive individuals can provide emotional support and help us navigate through challenging times. Participating in social activities, joining support groups, or seeking professional help can also be beneficial in managing stress effectively.

In conclusion, stress management plays a critical role in healthy aging. By incorporating regular physical activity, maintaining a balanced diet, practicing relaxation techniques, and nurturing a strong support system, we can effectively manage stress and promote overall well-being as we age. Remember, taking care of our mental and emotional health is just as important as taking care of our physical health in the journey towards longevity and healthy aging.

Quality Sleep and its Influence on Longevity

In our quest for healthy aging, one often overlooked yet vital component is quality sleep. As aging adults and health-conscious individuals, we understand the significance of a balanced diet and exercise, but we often underestimate the power of a good night's sleep. In this subchapter, we will delve into the profound influence that quality sleep can have on our longevity and overall well-being.

Sleep is a natural process that allows our bodies and minds to rejuvenate and repair themselves. It plays a crucial role in various aspects of our health, including cognitive function, immune system regulation, and emotional well-being. As we age, however, our sleep patterns tend to change, and obtaining a restful night's sleep becomes more challenging. This is why it becomes even more important for aging adults to prioritize quality sleep.

Research has shown that individuals who consistently get enough sleep have a lower risk of developing chronic health conditions such as heart disease, obesity, and diabetes. Additionally, quality sleep is closely linked to cognitive health, as it enhances memory retention and overall mental clarity. By prioritizing sleep, we can potentially reduce the risk of age- related cognitive decline and maintain sharper cognitive function as we age.

Furthermore, quality sleep plays a significant role in regulating our immune system. During sleep, our bodies produce and release cytokines, proteins that help combat inflammation and infection. By ensuring adequate sleep, we can enhance our immune response, protect ourselves from illnesses, and promote longevity.

To achieve quality sleep, it is essential to establish healthy sleep habits. This includes maintaining a consistent sleep schedule, creating a comfortable sleeping environment, and adopting relaxation techniques before bedtime. Additionally, avoiding stimulants such as caffeine and electronic devices close to bedtime can contribute to better sleep quality.

In conclusion, quality sleep is an integral part of healthy aging. As aging adults and health-conscious individuals, we must recognize its profound influence on our longevity and overall well-being. By prioritizing quality sleep and adopting healthy sleep habits, we can enhance our cognitive function, strengthen our immune system, and reduce the risk of chronic health conditions. So let us embrace the power of quality sleep and unlock the secrets of healthy aging.

Chapter 9: Strategies for Successful Long-Term Aging

Building a Support System

In the journey towards healthy aging, one of the crucial aspects that often gets overlooked is the importance of building a strong support system. As aging adults and health-conscious individuals, we must recognize that maintaining a healthy lifestyle and making dietary changes can be challenging without the right support network in place.

When it comes to nutrition for longevity, having a support system can make a world of difference. Surrounding yourself with like-minded individuals who are also committed to healthy aging can provide the necessary motivation and encouragement to stay on track. Whether it's joining a local health and wellness group, attending cooking classes, or participating in online forums, connecting with others who share similar goals can be incredibly beneficial.

Additionally, it's crucial to involve your loved ones in your journey towards healthy aging. Family and friends can play a significant role in supporting your dietary choices and lifestyle changes. By educating them about the importance of nutrition for longevity, you can gain their understanding and enlist their support. This might include inviting them to join you in meal planning and preparation, trying new recipes together, or simply having open conversations about your goals.

Another important aspect of building a support system is seeking professional guidance. Consulting with a registered dietitian or nutritionist who specializes in healthy aging can provide you with personalized recommendations and guidance tailored to your specific needs. They can help you create a well-balanced meal plan, navigate dietary restrictions, and address any concerns you may have.

Lastly, don't underestimate the power of self-support. Cultivating a positive mindset and practicing self-care are essential components of maintaining a healthy lifestyle. Engaging in activities that promote relaxation and stress reduction, such as meditation, yoga, or engaging hobbies, can contribute to overall well-being and support your longevity goals.

Remember, building a support system is not a one-time effort but an ongoing process. It requires proactive engagement, open communication, and a willingness to seek help when needed. By nurturing a strong support network, you can create an environment that fosters your healthy aging journey, ensuring long-term success and well-being.

In conclusion, building a support system is a vital component of nutrition for longevity. Surrounding yourself with like-minded individuals, involving your loved ones, seeking professional guidance, and practicing self-care are all essential elements of a robust support network. By harnessing the power of your support system, you can navigate the challenges of healthy aging with confidence and achieve optimal well- being.

Staying Motivated and Focused on Longevity Goals

As aging adults and health-conscious individuals, we all strive for a long and vibrant life. We want to maintain our energy, vitality, and overall well- being as we age gracefully. Achieving these goals requires not only adopting a healthy diet and lifestyle but also staying motivated and focused on our longevity objectives. In this subchapter, we will uncover effective strategies to help you stay on track and maintain your enthusiasm for healthy aging.

Setting clear and realistic goals is crucial for staying motivated. Start by identifying what you want to achieve in terms of your health and longevity. Do you want to lose weight, improve your energy levels, or reduce your risk of chronic diseases? Once you have defined your goals, break them down into smaller, achievable steps. This will not only make your objectives more manageable but also provide you with a sense of accomplishment along the way.

Accountability is another important factor in maintaining motivation. Find a partner or join a support group of like-minded individuals who share your goals. Having someone to hold you accountable and provide encouragement can significantly increase your chances of success.

Additionally, consider tracking your progress through a journal or mobile app to monitor your achievements and identify areas for improvement.

To stay focused on your longevity goals, it is essential to find purpose and meaning in your journey. Remind yourself regularly why you are striving for healthy aging. Perhaps you want to be an active grandparent, travel the world, or simply enjoy a high quality of life. Visualize these aspirations and connect them with your daily actions. This will help you stay motivated, especially during challenging times.

Another effective strategy is to celebrate your successes. Reward yourself for reaching milestones or sticking to your healthy habits. Treat yourself to a massage, indulge in a hobby you love, or spend quality time with loved ones. These rewards will reinforce your commitment to healthy aging and make the journey more enjoyable.

Lastly, remember to be kind to yourself. Setbacks and obstacles are natural, but it's crucial not to let them derail your progress. Instead of dwelling on mistakes, learn from them and move forward. Practice self- compassion and celebrate the small victories along the way.

By staying motivated and focused on your longevity goals, you are taking proactive steps towards a healthier and more fulfilling life. Embrace these strategies, find support, and maintain a positive mindset as you embark on this transformative journey of healthy aging.

Remember, the path to longevity is not a sprint but a marathon, and with dedication and perseverance, you can achieve your goals and enjoy the benefits of a vibrant and fulfilling life.

Celebrating Progress and Embracing Aging

Subchapter: Celebrating Progress and Embracing Aging

Introduction:

In the journey of life, aging is an inevitable process that every individual undergoes. However, embracing this natural progression is essential to living a fulfilling and meaningful life. In this subchapter, we will explore the concept of celebrating progress and embracing aging, particularly in the context of nutrition for longevity. By understanding the secrets of healthy aging and adopting the right diet and eating habits, aging adults and health-conscious individuals can unlock the potential for a vibrant and fulfilling life.

The Beauty of Progress:

As we age, it is crucial to celebrate the progress we have made throughout our lives. Each wrinkle, gray hair, and experience holds a unique story that contributes to our wisdom and character. By shifting our perspective and recognizing the beauty in these signs of aging, we can embrace the journey of life with gratitude and a sense of accomplishment.

Optimizing Nutrition for Healthy Aging:

Nutrition plays a pivotal role in healthy aging. The choices we make regarding our diet and eating habits can significantly impact our overall well-being and longevity. In this subchapter, we will delve into the best practices of nutrition for longevity, unveiling the secrets that can help us age gracefully and maintain optimal health.

The Power of a Balanced Diet:

A balanced diet is the foundation of healthy aging. Consuming a variety of nutrient-dense foods, including fruits, vegetables, whole grains, lean proteins, and healthy fats, provides the body with the necessary vitamins, minerals, and antioxidants to support cellular health, boost the immune system, and prevent chronic diseases commonly associated with aging.

Mindful Eating and Portion Control:

In addition to a balanced diet, mindful eating and portion control are crucial aspects of nutrition for longevity. By cultivating awareness and savoring each bite, we can enhance our digestion, prevent overeating, and foster a healthier relationship with food. Understanding portion sizes and listening to our body's hunger and satiety cues allow us to maintain a healthy weight and prevent age-related health issues.

The Role of Hydration:

Proper hydration is often underestimated but plays a vital role in healthy aging. As we age, our body's water content decreases, making it crucial to stay adequately hydrated. Drinking sufficient water throughout the day supports digestion, circulation, cognitive function, and overall cellular health.

Conclusion:

Celebrating progress and embracing aging are essential components of living a fulfilling and vibrant life. By adopting the secrets of healthy aging through optimal nutrition, we can enhance our physical, mental, and emotional well-being. With a balanced diet, mindful eating, portion control, and proper hydration, aging adults and health-conscious individuals can unlock the potential for longevity and vitality, savoring each moment of their journey.

Chapter 10: Conclusion

Recap of Key Concepts

As we come to the end of this chapter, let's take a moment to recap the key concepts discussed in "Eating for Longevity: Unveiling the Secrets of Healthy Aging." This book is dedicated to aging adults and health- conscious individuals who are seeking to optimize their nutrition for longevity and healthy aging.

Throughout this chapter, we have explored the concept of nutrition for longevity and discovered the best diet and eating habits for healthy aging. We have highlighted the importance of a balanced diet that incorporates a variety of nutrients, including lean proteins, whole grains, fruits, vegetables, and healthy fats. This balanced approach ensures that our bodies receive the necessary nutrients to support optimal health and aging.

One of the key takeaways from this chapter is the significance of maintaining a healthy weight. Excessive weight gain can increase the risk of chronic diseases such as heart disease, diabetes, and certain types of cancer. By implementing healthy eating habits and portion control, we can achieve and maintain a healthy weight, reducing the risk of these diseases and promoting longevity.

Another important concept we discussed is the role of antioxidants in our diet. Antioxidants are compounds found in fruits, vegetables, and whole grains that help protect our cells from damage caused by free radicals. By incorporating antioxidant-rich foods into our diet, we can combat the effects of aging and reduce the risk of age-related diseases.

We also emphasized the importance of hydration for healthy aging. Drinking an adequate amount of water throughout the day is essential for maintaining optimal bodily functions, improving digestion, and promoting healthier skin. Proper hydration also plays a crucial role in reducing the risk of certain age-related conditions such as urinary tract infections and constipation.

Lastly, we explored the benefits of regular physical activity in conjunction with a healthy diet. Engaging in regular exercise not only helps maintain a healthy weight but also improves overall cardiovascular health, strengthens bones and muscles, and enhances cognitive function. By incorporating both nutrition and exercise into our daily routines, we can enhance our chances of living a longer and healthier life.

In conclusion, this chapter has provided valuable insights into the best diet and eating habits for healthy aging. By

implementing these key concepts into our daily lives, we can

unlock the secrets of healthy aging and promote longevity.

Stay tuned for the next chapter, where we will delve deeper

into the specific foods and nutrients that support healthy aging.

Embracing a Lifelong Journey to Healthy Aging

As we age, our bodies go through various changes, and it becomes even more crucial to take care of our health and well-being. The key to healthy aging lies in adopting a holistic approach that encompasses not only physical well-being but also mental and emotional health. In this subchapter, we delve into the concept of embracing a lifelong journey to healthy aging, focusing on nutrition for longevity and discovering the best diet and eating habits for healthy aging.

For aging adults and health-conscious individuals, it is essential to understand that healthy aging is not a destination but a continuous process. It is about making conscious choices every day that contribute to your overall well-being. Nutrition plays a pivotal role in this journey, and by adopting the right dietary habits, you can significantly enhance your quality of life.

One of the secrets to healthy aging is consuming a well-balanced diet that is rich in nutrients. Opt for whole, unprocessed foods that provide essential vitamins, minerals, and antioxidants. Include a variety of fruits, vegetables, lean proteins, whole grains, and healthy fats in your meals. These foods help combat inflammation, boost your immune system, and provide the necessary fuel for your body to function optimally.

Another aspect of healthy aging is portion control. As we age, our metabolism slows down, making it easier to gain weight. By being mindful of portion sizes, you can maintain a healthy weight and reduce the risk of chronic diseases such as obesity, diabetes, and heart disease. Additionally, drinking plenty of water and staying hydrated is crucial for healthy aging, as it supports digestion, circulation, and overall cellular function.

Furthermore, it is important to pay attention to your eating habits and develop a positive relationship with food. Practice mindful eating by savoring each bite, eating slowly, and listening to your body's hunger and fullness cues. Avoid emotional eating and seek healthier coping mechanisms for stress and other emotional challenges.

Lastly, a lifelong journey to healthy aging involves staying physically active and engaging in regular exercise. Find activities that you enjoy and that align with your abilities. Whether it's walking, swimming, yoga, or strength training, staying active not only improves physical health but also enhances cognitive function and mental well-being.

Embracing a lifelong journey to healthy aging requires dedication, consistency, and a commitment to self-care. By adopting a nutritious diet, practicing mindful eating, staying physically active, and nurturing your mental and emotional health, you can unlock the secrets of healthy aging and enjoy a vibrant and fulfilling life as you grow older. Remember, it's never too late to start, and every small step towards better health counts on this journey.

Final Thoughts and Words of Encouragement

As we conclude our journey through the pages of "Eating for Longevity: Unveiling the Secrets of Healthy Aging," we want to leave you with some final thoughts and words of encouragement. Aging adults and health- conscious individuals seeking to improve their nutrition for longevity are taking a significant step towards a healthier and more fulfilling life. Remember, it is never too late to make positive changes and embrace a lifestyle that supports healthy aging.

Throughout this book, we have explored the secrets of healthy aging, delving into the best diet and eating habits that can extend our years and enhance our well-being. We have learned that a balanced and nutrient- rich diet, coupled with regular physical activity, is the foundation for healthy aging. By focusing on whole foods, such as fruits, vegetables, whole grains, lean proteins, and healthy fats, we can provide our bodies with the vital nutrients they need to thrive.

However, it is important to remember that no diet is one-size-fits-all. Each person has unique nutritional needs, so it is crucial to listen to your body and adapt your eating habits accordingly. Pay attention to how different foods make you feel and make adjustments as needed. Consult with a healthcare professional or registered dietitian to develop a personalized nutrition plan that aligns with your specific needs and goals.

While nutrition is undoubtedly a key factor in healthy aging, it is just one piece of the puzzle. Nurturing our mental and emotional well-being is equally important. Surround yourself with positive influences, engage in activities that bring you joy, and practice stress-reducing techniques such as meditation or mindfulness. Remember, aging is a natural process, and it is essential to embrace it with grace and gratitude.

In conclusion, aging adults and health-conscious individuals hold the power to shape their own destinies when it comes to healthy aging. By adopting a nutrient-rich diet, engaging in regular physical activity, and nurturing our mental and emotional well-being, we can unlock the secrets of healthy aging and enjoy a longer, more fulfilling life. So, go forth with confidence and make the choices that will nourish your body, mind, and spirit, allowing you to embrace the gift of longevity and live life to the fullest.